I0447103

Fibromyalgia: My Journey from Depression to Dancing

Christine Weston, Ph.D.

I dedicate this book to my family and thank them for their support as I went through this difficult process. I would especially like to recognize my brother, Ted, who always believed in my abilities although he never understood them. Rest in peace, my brother. You will always be remembered.

Introduction

My journey with fibromyalgia began many years ago, although my diagnosis did not occur until 2003. This book provides insights into my process starting with living unknowingly with the syndrome and continuing through my diagnosis, research, and ultimately my path to recovery. The first part of the book focuses on my experience and some of the insights I have gleaned from living with fibro and being in remission. The second part of the book focuses on the information that I applied to my healing process as I earned my Ph.D. in Holistic Health.

Part 1 My Journey

Introduction to Fibromyalgia

What is Fibromyalgia?

Fibromyalgia, commonly referred to as "fibro" is a syndrome, recognized by the medical community since the early 1990's. The name fibromyalgia describes the syndrome, which encompasses several specific symptoms. The symptoms include but are not limited to chronic-wide-spread pain (in all four quadrants of the body), chronic fatigue, unclear or "foggy" thinking, depression, bladder infections, spastic colons and lower back pain.

Fibro is diagnosed by eliminating other conditions such as Lupus, through blood tests, and then checking tender points (18 points on the body that when touched cause severe pain on people with fibro). Most doctors also administer the Fibromyalgia Impact Questionnaire (FIQ) as part of the diagnosis. The patient answers 10 questions regarding pain, depression and quality of life.

The doctor then scores the FIQ and incorporates this score into the diagnosis.

Confirmation of the diagnosis occurs when at least 11 of the 18 points are positive for pain and certain pain conditions are present. These conditions include: the pain must have lasted more than three months, it must occur in all four quadrants of the body and it usually is not stationary, meaning it may hurt in one place on one day and another the next day. The doctor usually performs some blood and other diagnostic tests to eliminate the other diseases, but usually, if the person has pain on 11 of the points, has pain on all four quadrants of the body and has had the pain for more than 3 months, the diagnosis is certain.

Other conditions usually accompany fibro, such as chronic fatigue, depression and fibro fog. One of the problems with diagnosing fibro is that many of the symptoms can exist on their own. For example, chronic fatigue can be a stand-alone diagnosis. People can have chronic fatigue without having fibromyalgia, but people with fibro generally experience chronic fatigue. Similarly, depression can and often does exist without being part of fibro, but most people diagnosed with fibro include depression and/or anxiety as part of their symptoms.

Fibro patients also have constant, unrelenting pain. The best way to describe the pain is that it is flu-like. Everything hurts, constantly. The muscles and bone constantly ache. Relief from pain is elusive at best.

Each of the conditions mentioned above works together to exacerbate the pain and each condition exacerbates all of the others. As a person becomes more depressed, he/she becomes more tired. As the fatigue increases, the person moves less. As movement decreases, pain increases. As pain increases, the ability to think clearly diminishes. As clear thinking decreases, depression increases. A downward spiral condition occurs that is extremely difficult to break. Breaking out of that spiral is the key to creating a life and really living again, even with fibro.

The medical community, at the time I was diagnosed and looking for treatment, considered fibro a condition would flare up and then recede. In other words, there were times when you had some pain and times when you had a LOT of pain. This was not my experience. My experience was constant, significant pain at the level of about 8 out of 10 almost every day.

Having gone through my healing processes, I now know that the cyclical nature of the syndrome kept me locked into increasing pain, diminished mental capacity, and increased depression. The medical community does not necessarily realize or acknowledge that these cycles occur or are relevant. More often, the symptoms are considered and/or are treated separately and are not considered holistically. In my opinion the symptoms must be considered as part of the whole and must be addressed simultaneously.

A little perspective about fibromyalgia would probably be good. Fibro seems to be the new buzzword, the new disease to have after eliminating everything else. Many people who suffer from the syndrome have sought medical treatment for a number of the symptoms, only to be told that there is "nothing wrong" because fibro is difficult to diagnose. It has baffled the medical community for a long time.

No one knows where it comes from and certainly no one knows how to fix it... though many believe that they do. The "experts" that I met all provided different treatment plans designed to fix fibro. They were all sure they are right and, unfortunately, the plans were all different and often contradictory. To make matters worse, none of the people that I have met, who claim to know how to fix it, have actually experienced fibro

themselves, so their perspectives are much different than

the perspective of someone who lives with it, day in and

day out. It is my intention to provide an insider's look at

how the syndrome progresses and how to alleviate some

of the symptoms.

Although my doctors, nurses, chronic pain team

and other providers meant well and attempted to treat

my syndrome, my experience is that they did not have

the appropriate tools or information to provide effective

treatment. Some of the suggestions from the medical

community were amazing and did offer temporary relief,

such as yoga, swimming, and meditation, but some of

the others, including significant medications, did not help

to resolve the issue.

The approaches/remedies that have worked for

me include breaking the pain cycle, learning how to

obtain deep sleep, losing weight, and eliminating or

reducing stress. I have integrated quite a few methodologies into breaking the cycles, but making changes in these areas were the key to unchaining from fibro.

What Fibro is Not

One of the most important thing to consider when looking at what fibro is not would be to emphasize that it is not a figment of anyone's imagination. I know that it is tempting to think that something like this is just some sort of "psychosomatic" problem and dismiss it at that. While I believe that the psyche significantly influences the physical body, the term psychosomatic is often interpreted as derogatory, indicating that the person is making up the problem or condition.

Disease starts somewhere. In my experience and in my belief system, it results from a lesson that we are supposed to learn in this lifetime. The second part of this book details exactly how the various levels of our body work together to create dis-ease at the physical level. Briefly it means if we are able to resolve the lesson while it is still out in the outer layers of our body, we usually do not fall ill. If, however, we are not able to resolve the problem it manifests closer and closer to our physical body. One of the layers of the body is the mental layer, so in that sense, yes, all disease is psychosomatic, or having to do with our mental processing.

So, ok, it is psychosomatic, to one extent or another as are all diseases and illnesses. This does not mean that a person who has fibro has chosen, at a conscious level, to bring in this syndrome. It simply means that they were not able to resolve the problem at the mental or other layers, so it manifested physically. This does not mean it is their fault, and it certainly does not mean that they are sick on purpose. It means that it has manifested in a physical way in order to be dealt with on a physical level. The outer layers must be dealt with also in order to bring about long term or permanent relief. Much more about these theories in part 2!

Who is affected by Fibromyalgia and What are the Costs?

Fibromyalgia is much more than a catch all for vague unspecific symptoms. It is a real health problem affecting millions of people in our country and around the world.

According to the National Fibromyalgia Association (NFA), approximately 10 million Americans and between 3 and 6% of the world population have this syndrome (2011). Far more women than men have been diagnosed (75-90%), which is not to say that more women than men have it, just that they have been diagnosed. There are a number of reasons for this disparity including the fact that women tend to visit doctors more and tend to be more receptive to medical (or alternative) treatment. The usual diagnosis occurs between 20 and 50 years of age. Older people have a higher occurrence of fibro and it affects approximately 8% of the over 80 population (NFA, 2011).

For each person that has fibro at least one other person (usually more like 2 or 3) is affected in some way. This might mean taking the person to the doctor occasionally or being a shoulder to cry on or it could involve full-time round the clock care for the fibro patient. The associated costs are very high, with an estimated $12-14 billion US expenditure per year on fibro. This represents between 1-2% of the nation's productivity. The NFA indicates that the annual medical costs for people with fibro are twice as high as they are for other people. It also indicates that the level of disability for people with fibro is twice as high as for people who do not have it. Employers spend approximately $50-100 in indirect costs for every dollar spent on fibro. Interestingly, the NFA also indicates that people who suffer from fibro are twice as likely to use alternative and complementary medicines (2011).

This syndrome does not exist in a vacuum. It is significant health problem, which affects millions of lives day in and day out and places a heavy financial burden on the patients, the families and the employers.

My Experience with Fibro

Quality of Life

My energy level has always been very high and I have always been able to accomplish just about anything I set my sights on. Although some physical problems occurred here and there, for the most part, I did not let circumstances or my health get in the way of my doing whatever I wanted. My life was never static, but always changing and morphing as I embraced the newest project, career advancement, educational goal, or move from one house, apartment, city or state to another.

Prior to having children, I was always on the go. If there was a dance, a conference or any other social event of interest within driving distance, I usually attended. If an event occurred that was more than 5 or 6 hours away, I would plan a road trip. Driving 2 hours to

Monterey to watch a sunrise on the spur of the moment was not out of the question. Once, a friend of mine and I decided to go to a conference in Yosemite (about 4 hours away). We threw some things into suitcases, drove like crazy, hung out with friends for a couple of hours and then decided we really wanted to go to a dance in Orinda, so we headed back and caught the end of the dance. I loved my independence and ability to do whatever I wanted to do.

During the years before the kids were born, I worked in a variety of jobs, including retail, door-to-door, and telephone sales, photography, and waitressing. I realized that these jobs were not going to help me on a career path so I continually attended two or three classes at a time, at the local community colleges. I never gave up the dream of having a college education, even though I did not attend college full time for my lower division work.

My energy began to wane a little bit in my late 20's, when a series of events took the wind out of my sails. The first event involved the death of a gentleman I had recently started dating. Although we were only together a short time, I had fallen for him in a way that I had never fallen previously. He died riding his motorcycle, on his way to meet me at a dance. His death shook me to the foundations and altered everything in my life. I was an emotional wreck for many years, which affected every area of my life. For several months, I contemplated suicide almost daily. Eventually I moved into my father's house, so I wouldn't take my life.

As I was pulling out of this despair, I started to date another friend of mine. His life was a mess and he broached the subject of making a suicide pact. I had just past the brink of wanting to die, and tried to convince him that he could survive his pain and that the feelings would pass. He was unconvinced and not long afterward, he shot himself.

I believe that the deaths of these two men were catalysts for major turning points in my life including the exacerbation of pain and depression and the beginning of fibro. Depression and despair accompanied me wherever I went, although I was able to maintain outward composure much of the time. After their deaths, I made several rapid life changes. I dated several men, eventually became pregnant, lost the baby and then became pregnant again. I quickly married, had the baby, had another baby and then divorced. I lived a nightmare life where change occurred rapidly and without much thought of consequences. Mostly, I wanted to ease the pain of the deaths.

The tactics that I chose to kill pain didn't work very effectively. I wanted to not feel the pain, but I don't drink or take recreational drugs, so food seemed like a good option. During my pregnancies I gained a considerable amount of weight. The kids were born 14 months apart, and the miscarriage occurred just a few months before my daughter's pregnancy, so my body didn't have time to recover from one pregnancy before it started in on the next and then the next. I always experienced back pain, from accidents when I was a kid, but suddenly the pain was exacerbated from the pregnancies and the extra weight. I don't remember experiencing other physical pain at this time, but the lower back pain, weight gain, emotional despair, and depression were constant. Although I had always been tiny prior to getting pregnant, I found myself unable to shed the extra weight. In fact, it kept increasing over the years. Eventually I topped out at 244 pounds. Part of my fibro recovery journey has included losing the excess weight.

Not long after my son's birth, in 1989, my ex-husband and I split up for the last time (we were married less than 2 years). I found myself alone with 2 toddlers and no particular skills. I had always managed to make a living, but I wanted to do more with my life and set a good example for the kids. I especially wanted a college degree, so I finished my Associate in Arts and headed off to UC Berkeley. My Berkeley experience differed from most undergraduates. Most of the people I went to school with lived on campus, were in their late teens or early 20s, and socialized around school, hanging out in coffee shops or sororities.

I was in my early 30s, my daughter turned three the day before I started classes, and my son turned two shortly thereafter. I worked as a research assistant and had another job or two on campus. Sometimes I had to travel for my main job, so I was out of town here and there. The daycare at Berkeley was a cooperative so I was required to do some volunteer work every week. I didn't have any time for hanging around on campus or with my friends. I was a single mom, with two toddlers and two or three jobs attempting to earn a degree from one of the most prestigious universities in the world! It was quite an undertaking. I ended up graduating with honors!

Sometime after finishing Berkeley, my body really started to slow down. I continued to work several jobs at a time until I obtained my corporate position, but I was chronically fatigued. I was cranky and I did not have energy to play or to do much else. I worked and I slept. My kids ached for me to play with them but I was short tempered, overweight, and I suffered from migraines. I'm sure that my lack of patience and my migraines were direct results of the increase in weight, stress, depression, and pain.

Eventually I landed a wonderful position, managing syndicated research at Wells Fargo Bank. This meant that I commuted 50 miles to work since I lived first in Sonoma County then in Contra Costa County, while working in San Francisco. It also meant the end of juggling multiple jobs as I earned enough at this one position to take care of my family's needs. It felt like my career was on track and I focused much of my attention on the career and increasing responsibilities there.

One of the benefits of my new career included tuition assistance. My boss and I looked over a variety of Masters Programs and finally decided on an online MBA from the University of Phoenix. From 1998 until 2002, I added school back into my hectic schedule. I believe my fibro kicked into gear at this point, although I didn't realize it at the time.

During the years just prior to and after diagnosis, I spent a great deal of time sleeping and trying minimize pain. I was depressed and having panic attacks and didn't know how to stop them. I would lose thoughts, words and directions. I would avoid going places like the movies or grocery shopping because it hurt too much to stand or walk. Cleaning the house was a monstrous task that took several days to accomplish. I would estimate how much pain I would experience based on which activity I wanted to accomplish. Sometimes I could either vacuum or mop, but I could never even attempt both the same day. Going to a movie or a play was impossible most of the time because I couldn't sit in a chair long enough to get through the performance. I had occasional times where I was up to some recreational activity, but that meant significantly more time in bed the next day.

Because I telecommuted, I was able to hide most of my symptoms from my co-workers. Eventually, I approached my boss and told her about my physical condition. I had been an exemplary employee for many years, so her solution was for me to have a stack of books by my bed and to read the books on the days when I could not work. She knew that no matter what I would accomplish my tasks, and so she allowed me the freedom to work at my own pace. It was a great relief to me that she had that kind of faith in me. I never did put the stack of books by my bed, but I would take naps most days in between working stints.

The most difficult work days were those when I had to travel. I worked in an office based in San Francisco for several years. During the time I worked in SF, I lived first in Rohnert Park, CA (Sonoma County), then Oakley, CA (Contra Costa County), then Port Orchard, Washington. On the days I went to the office, I always had at least an hour and a half commute. If my day consisted of a meeting or two I generally did pretty well, because I could rest at a Starbucks on the way in to the meeting and immediately leave for home right afterward. The days where I had to actually work at the office were very challenging because the pain levels would increase as the day wore on. I usually left by 2:00 or 3:00 in the afternoon. I would then go home and sleep for a few hours, then get up and work for a while longer. If I had to travel to a meeting, I would make sure to arrive a day early and leave a day after the meeting, so I would have time to recover from sitting in the meeting. All-day trainings were absolute torture.

In short, I was a wreck most of the time, but it had been a gradual transition, so I integrated the changes as they arose and I figured I was normal; that I was just getting older and that everyone went through the pain that I was experiencing. Every now and then I'd have a good, more or less functional day and I would think that I was fine, so I would work really hard, get a lot of stuff done around the house and then would collapse again, exhausted.

I kept my symptoms to myself as much as possible. My son had gone to live with his dad so he was spared a lot of the anguish of this time, but my daughter lived with me and saw my pain every day. I was able to hide the panic attacks from her, but not the depression or the pain. The kids knew that I was tired all the time and had been since they were little. They resented this fact, and that I didn't feel good most of the time.

Until my mom made a comment about someone who was my age and barely able to get up or down the stairs, I didn't really realize how badly my health had declined, because the decline had been gradual. Mom indicated that it wasn't normal to not be able to go up and down stairs at 45 years old and that I should get checked out. So I did. I went to the doctor and got

diagnosed. Fibromyalgia; it sounded like the end of my

life.

Symptoms and Diagnosis

I didn't know that I was sick for a long time. Fibro snuck up on me, taking away a little more of my mobility and energy every year. One of the theories about the causes of fibro includes the possibility that traumatic events act as a catalyst. For me, the traumatic events included severe relationship challenges culminating in a move to Washington. I had lived in Washington many years earlier and loved its beauty and serenity. I maintained my position at Wells Fargo as my boss allowed me to telecommute.

The symptoms, which gradually emerged for me, included depression, widespread constant pain, panic attacks and fibro fog. I'd always had lower back pain and was used to dealing with it so I didn't really think of that pain as related to other pain. I had experienced several traumatic personal events in the recent past, so I figured my depression and panic attacks were due to circumstances, never realizing that they related to the fibro. I hadn't ever experienced anything like the fibro fog and it was extremely scary for me. I depended on my brain for my work and fun; to have it inaccessible was a new and frightening experience.

One interesting theory is that trauma brings on fibro and I'm quite sure events in my then recent past exacerbated the symptoms and perhaps brought on the full-fledged syndrome. I was date-raped in 2001, just before moving up to WA. Often it is a sexual trauma or an accident that acts as a catalyst for full-fledged fibro. I believe that in my case it was the straw that broke the proverbial camel's back.

By late 2002-2003 I found that I was having panic attacks and depression almost all the time. My pain level had increased so much that it was difficult for me to walk up and down the stairs and I was avoiding things like the grocery store and AA meetings (I've been in recovery, continuously sober, since 1978). I had frequent bouts of fibro-fog, which included forgetting things and very out of character occurrences like getting lost on the way to pick my daughter up from the airport. I frequently lost words and the ability to think critically.

I was able to work because I telecommuted and wasn't held to regular work hours. My boss knew that I could absolutely be counted on to get the job done, and I always did it well although it was often done in-between fibro-fog, panic attack, or depression spells. I didn't let anyone at work know how badly I was feeling because I didn't want them to feel sorry for me or think that I wasn't up to doing my job. Because my boss trusted me fully and allowed me to work my own hours, I was able to function.

Often my work was the thing that would get me out of bed and moving in the morning. I HAD to check my e-mail and I had to deliver a certain amount of work every day or I would fall further and further behind. So I would check it, attend any meetings (by phone) I needed to, call vendors and clients, and then go back to bed. For the most part, I was able to manage work around my illness and was able to wait to send critical e-mails until I was emotionally and mentally up to the task. I had an amazing assistant, who helped me keep all of the balls up in the air.

One of the key problems that I experienced was the inability to fall into a deep sleep. Because I was depressed and in pain, I would have thoughts and/or pain that would keep me awake most of the night. If I started to fall asleep, I would wake up because I was afraid my body would get hurt more while I was sleeping. If I weren't in the middle of a painful episode, I would often experience racing thoughts that would keep me awake. The end-result was the same; I was tired all the time. What is fascinating to look back on is that I had been tired, actually exhausted, for many years. I wasn't

getting the sleep my body required, so I never fully

rested.

The pain-depression-fatigue-fibro fog cycle was in

full swing during this time. Each symptom exacerbated

each other symptom until I felt like my body consisted of

nothing but pain and fatigue. I experienced almost

constant depression and anxiety, although I didn't

realize it until I pulled out of the cycle. What's really

interesting is that I was able to hold down a mid- level,

very visible position at one of the world's leading

financial institutions and be highly productive in my job,

while in the midst of this pain and turmoil.

In 2003, my doctors diagnosed me with

Fibromyalgia. I knew very little about fibro except that a

good friend of mine had it and she was convinced that I

had it also. What I did know was that my body hurt and I

was having trouble walking down the stairs in the

morning, tasks such as organizing my thoughts could be difficult, and exhaustion and depression were frequent companions. Other symptoms I experienced included anxiety, and weight gain. It had not occurred to me that these symptoms might exist as part of a comprehensive syndrome or that relief was possible. I thought I was just getting older and the natural consequence of aging included physical problems. In 2003, I was 45 years old.

At about the same time that my fried with fibro suggested I visit a doctor, a friend who is a nurse indicated that she thought I had it also, so I went to the doctor to get a professional opinion. The doctor conducted several tests (including a battery of blood tests) that eliminated diseases with similar symptoms, such as Lupus. Based on the test results, the doctor concluded I had fibro, and with that diagnosis my journey into the world of fibromyalgia began.

Upon arriving home from the doctor's office I started looking into the "syndrome" that I suddenly "had". At the time, I earned my living managing market research, so I dedicated several hours over the next week or so to researching fibro. I searched the web, found discussion groups, bought books, talked to a number of people who were already on the fibro path and spent a significant amount of time trying to determine the consequences of having this syndrome in my life.

One of the first things I realized is that I had been experiencing fibro symptoms for several years. I frequently dealt with excessive pain throughout my body, chronic fatigue, depression, bladder infections, fibro fog, and memory lapses. The thought that I was a hypochondriac had haunted me and it was liberating to realize this was not the case as all of these symptoms were part of the fibromyalgia syndrome. I was relieved to hear that a medical diagnosis for my symptoms existed. I often feared that the pain was psychosomatic or I convinced myself that I just needed to catch up on sleep and I would be fine.

Although I experienced depression prior to conducting my research due to the symptoms and life challenges that accompany the syndrome, significantly MORE depression set in after exploring the fibro world for a while. It seemed like the people who were in the chat rooms talking about fibro and sharing their day-to-day experiences had lives that were essentially over. They weren't able to do anything, except watch TV and they weren't always up to watching TV!!! I had been very discouraged prior to exploring this world, but I was significantly more depressed after a few days' research.

I'd like to say that my immediate attitude was that I would beat or manage fibro, but what I did instead was to go deeper into depression as I realized that my life, as

I knew it, was over. My perception was that people who had fibro were seldom able to continue working at their jobs, their ability to move was restricted, and they were in endless cycles of pain and fatigue. At that time, my body was in similar shape. I hurt so badly most of the time that I wanted to crawl into a hole and die. I could function at a minimal level for a short time, but any prolonged activity was out of the question.

Early in my time after diagnosis, I talked to one of my mother's friends who had been living with fibro for several years and she gave me a little hope. She found that with the right medications she was able to do things like dance again. I had a hard time believing I would ever walk easily again, much less dance, but I was encouraged by her words. Most of my responses to anyone introducing hopeful information about fibro were negative, because I did not believe there was any solution. The people in the chat rooms and forums had made it very clear that fibro was a one way street, all downhill, and that there was no hope in sight.

My path from there to here has been a long one, filled with research, additional education, financial loss, liberation and at last, a sense of peace and loss of pain. I no longer consider myself a person with fibro, although I do know that the symptoms can come back if I move back into unhealthy cycles.

Several years after diagnosis, my life is much different than it was when I was diagnosed. Today, I am pain free most of the time. I dance. I don't dance often or for long periods of time, but I dance. I thought that world was closed to me, but I find today that it is opening up very gently. I take it easy much of the time but I am determined to have a life again. For me that includes gardening, walking on the beach, taking photographs, swimming, writing, thinking, traveling, working and yes, dancing.

My message to those who have fibro is that you can have a life again. It isn't easy, it isn't always fun, but there is hope that you can be more than the person on the couch or in the bed reeling from pain watching your life slip away day by day.

Research and Treatment Options

When I was diagnosed I started looking into treatment options. I had dabbled in things like homeopathy over the years and I had become a pretty good energy worker by then. This means I helped people heal, by directing energy into the various levels of their bodies. I used Reiki and other healing methods. However, I immediately forgot everything I knew about holistic approaches and went off in search of medical solutions.

To my very great surprise, my doctor recommended things like massage, yoga, meditation and warm-water swimming. I thought she would start with medications and work upward from there, so I was very happily put back on the path of holistic wellness, right from the start.

One of the things I was convinced was affecting me was the weather. I was living in Washington State, having moved there about 2 years earlier from California. The weather is much colder in WA and I thought perhaps this was the reason I had developed fibro. It was a big enough certainty in my opinion, that I sold my house and moved back to CA. I was partly right and partly not right. The move back to CA didn't have any effect on my fibro, as I was still symptomatic, but as I get better I realize that the cold weather can sometimes still brings out symptoms, even though I'm in remission.

While I still lived in Washington I tried warm water swimming. It seemed to help while I was in the pool, if the water was warm enough, but I started the swimming during the winter. Any positive affect that I realized from the water was negated by the walk back to the car in the cold! The cold weather caused my muscles to clinch, which immediately undid any relaxation I had experienced in the warm water.

Once I made it back to CA, I made sure to set up an appointment with someone who was assuredly a fibro specialist. During our first appointment, I realized this was really not true. His only response to my questions about how to treat fibro was to tell me there wasn't anything to do about it, but if I insisted he'd send me to a rheumatologist. I was pretty disenchanted with the doctor and since it was just about time for open enrollment at our company, I decided to change my coverage. I switched back to Kaiser and went to see someone there about the fibro.

My experiences with Kaiser were tremendous. They not only have classes on fibro and chronic pain, they have a chronic pain team that works with people to teach patients how to have some semblance of a normal life. I didn't get referred there right away; however, I had to go the long way around! I mentioned my fibro to my nurse practitioner, but didn't make a big deal about it so we didn't really attack it until 2005. I spent 2004 in tremendous pain, feeling like there weren't really any solutions. I did work with my acupuncturist a little bit, but other than that I just lived in pain.

My fibro is exacerbated by chronic back pain. In addition, in July 2005, I was in an auto accident (I was rear-ended), so I attempted to fix the damage from the accident first. I went to Kaiser several times to figure out how to deal with this new upper back pain. I had been given a nice combination of soma and a muscle relaxer right after the accident. They took away ALL of my pain!!! I was so excited. I hadn't been pain free for so many years I couldn't believe that I found the answer. I went to my doctor and asked her to refill both the prescriptions. She said no & that these pills were very addictive. I told her I didn't care. I was finally pain free and wanted to keep taking them. I'm sure it was difficult for her, but she refused to give them to me.

I stopped seeing the doctor and acupuncturist (also at Kaiser) and went to my chiropractor instead. We had some success early on with dealing with the initial pain through manipulations, massage and heat. He took my healing as far as he could and then sent me back to Kaiser after a few months. Because the damage from the accident had exacerbated the back AND fibro conditions so much, my doctor took me off of work and had me start working with the chronic pain team.

The team did an in-depth diagnosis, which lasted 4 hours. They had me visit a pharmacologist, a psychiatrist, a pain specialist and a physical therapist in one visit. This team then consulted on my case and decided I had fibromyalgia, high-blood pressure, depression and some disc degeneration. They recommended that I have some sort of treatment for depression and work with my doctor on drug therapies for my fibro. I was then sent to the chronic pain and fibro classes.

I was very willing to start taking narcotics although I have been in recovery for many years. My doctor again felt like we should put off any narcotic treatment for as long as possible, for which I am very grateful. Instead, we used muscle relaxers and a strong anti-inflammatory. I was to take up to 6 of each every day. At that time I would usually end up taking 5 of each a day. (At the time of this writing I rarely take any muscle relaxers or pain relievers).

I never did return to my job as the daily pain stayed with me for another year and a half. By then I had started my holistic store and was seeking alternative remedies for alleviating the pain.

The fibro and chronic pain classes at Kaiser taught some great information, but they also missed a few points. They were wonderful about teaching acupressure points, sleep habits, journaling pain and enlisting help. The parts that they missed concerned the difference between flare-ups and chronic pain, how to deal with the fog, and what chronic pain actually felt like. The practitioners had no personal experience in this area and did not have a sense of how it felt to always be in pain, so they couldn't really grasp that there wasn't a formula. They taught that there were certain things that we did that caused the pain, therefore if we avoided those things we wouldn't have pain or flare ups. This is a critical error in their teaching and assumptions. I, like all of my classmates, experienced non-stop pain rather than flare-ups.

My Path to Recovery

As previously indicated, one of the treatments that was highly recommended for muscle relaxation was warm water swimming. When I moved back to CA, I bought a house with a small pool. The pool had a "spa" setting and I could warm it up to 95 degrees (or higher). This helped me to relax although I remained very sick and steadily worsening for the first year after I moved home. In the summer of 2005, when I was rear ended, the accident exacerbated the symptoms and caused some damage to my mid and upper back. I had always experienced lower back pain, but the new pain was in between my shoulders in the middle of my back. Along with the new back pain, I experienced even more extreme fatigue.

My work day shifted significantly about the same time. I had telecommuted for a long time, but we suddenly had a boss who was not a fan of distance work. He wanted us in the office all of the time. So, instead of being able to deal with my illness at home and work around the pain, I had to be in San Francisco every day. I used public transportation as much as possible, but this meant standing on the BART platform in the cold, the ride on the train which jolted me around and then a 15 minute walk to the office in the biting, windy cold of downtown San Francisco. I decided to go in early and drive instead.

The memories of those last months at Wells Fargo are a nightmare. My pain and depression were at an all-time high. I could barely function, much less be an active participant in my kids' lives. My son was living with us because his Dad was stationed in Iraq for a year. My daughter was very angry with me for moving her from one high school to another between her sophomore and junior years. Neither of the kids was doing very well and I didn't have any energy to help them through this critical time. Working and pain management were taking all of my energy.

I managed my life very carefully in those last Wells Fargo days. I would arrive in the office around 6:30 so I would miss the traffic. I'd walk across the parking lot in tears because the ground hurt my feet so badly from fibro pain. Soon after arriving, after checking e-mail, I would take a nap in the library, before anyone else arrived. I'd get up and work for a couple of hours, then usually have my first melt down due to back pain around 10 or 11 am. I'd sleep again for an hour or so if I could and then work for a couple more hours. By 2:00 I'd be in total meltdown, having taken any number of pain medications (over the counter), which didn't relieve my symptoms much, but took a little of the edge off. I'd leave, drive home, sleep for a bit and then work for several more hours.

I kept this pattern up for about 8 months. My new boss didn't really know that I was sick as I was determined to keep it from him, not wanting him to feel sorry for me or to keep assignments from me because of my condition. Eventually, around Christmas of 2005 I told him I had fibro and that was the reason I telecommuted as much as possible. He had no idea that I was sick because I was able to manage my pain pretty well.

Searching for Alternatives

Eventually, in March of 2006 my doctor took me off of work. I had reached an all-time high of pain, my blood pressure and weight were very high and I was hardly able to string two thoughts together. Stopping work to me was very scary. I thought that I would end up like the people that I had read about when I was first diagnosed. They were unable to do anything, were on disability, couldn't function and were just about bed ridden. I was afraid that I would end up like that.

Instead, this was the beginning of the healing cycle for me. I was able to sleep enough because I bought a good bed when I moved back to CA and I finally had time to relax. I started to take care of myself a little bit. I hadn't realized that I had stopped doing little things like painting my fingernails years before. I had stopped paying attention to my body. My body had been yelling at me for years to listen to it, but I was too busy and in too much pain to hear it. The busier I became, the harder my body tried to get my attention. The more it tried to get my attention, the more I tried to push it away. I was in deep emotional, spiritual and physical pain and I had no idea how to break out of it. Stopping work meant that I stopped running away from pain.

For the first few months I didn't do a lot. It took all of my energy to get out of the house and go to the grocery store. One errand, sometimes two in a day were all that I could manage. I spent most of my time at home on the couch with friends coming to visit and check in on me. I had a huge number of doctor appointments, trying to confirm the diagnosis of my conditions and figure out how to deal with them.

Fortunately I was with Kaiser. Kaiser has a great chronic pain department and really good tools to help people work with their pain. The first thing they did was put me through the 4 hour diagnosis with 4 or 5 practitioners. As I mentioned, the team consisted of a physical therapist, a chronic pain doctor, a psychiatrist and a pharmacologist. Each spent quite a bit of time talking to me, diagnosing the problems and figuring out an approach that would incorporate all of their diagnoses. They determined that yes, I really did have fibro, but I also had degenerative disc disease (exacerbated by the accident), depression, and high blood pressure.

The recommendations from the pain team were to work with my doctor on medications, attend the chronic pain and fibro classes and work on the depression. They didn't recommend counseling, although I wish they had because I think that would have been beneficial for me. I have been in recovery since 1978 so my doctor didn't want me to go on any of the narcotics that many fibro patients take. By the time the doctors were recommending narcotics, I was unwilling to take them, so I was never hooked into that cycle. For that I am eternally grateful.

A few months after this diagnosis when I was still fighting to get disability from my insurance carrier (I never did get it after the first month), I decided to start working on my Ph.D. I had been considering this for several years, as I found a school that offered a Ph.D. in Philosophy in Metaphysics. I had always been interested in metaphysics and was a Reiki Master, but I felt this wasn't quite what I was looking for. About the time I seriously considered going after this degree, the school that I had wanted to attend suddenly had a new Ph.D. in Holistic Health. I knew this was the program for me and I signed up for it immediately.

By now it was September of 2006. I had pretty well figured out that I wasn't going to be able to go back to my job. My pain was still significant, my fatigue level was very high and I had constant brain fog. I was able to grasp many of the concepts in the degree work, but some of them took a really long time to sink in. The work was self-paced so I was able to get through it when I could think and let it go when I couldn't.

A friend of mine approached me about starting a business and I jumped on the idea. It was to create a salon and a new age book store with an art gallery. She hit all of my hot buttons with the art gallery and new age bookstore. I was intrigued and we started tossing around the idea of opening a business. The deal we made was that I would do the financial end and she would for the most part run it. I'd be around some but my health was so bad I was afraid to commit to being an active participant. This shifted pretty quickly as we moved from ideas to action.

I was very interested in letting go of the pain/fatigue/depression cycle and started implementing changes to cut through it. The changes I had to make were all about figuring out how to sleep enough so the pain would lessen. I had to start swimming at night in my warm (90+ degrees) pool to get my muscles moving. I had to buy a bed that wasn't two mattresses on the floor, but was something that would support me. I had to make changes so that I could function.

The Process of Letting Fibro Go

When I began work on my Ph.D., I had no idea that my studies would turn into a journey of self-exploration. I thought I was going to get the degree to add some sort of legitimacy to the healing work that had intrigued me for years. I have known I'm a gifted healer for a long time, and have taken numerous classes in the pursuit of figuring out exactly what that means and how I can apply it to my life and help the people around me. Going after a degree in holistic health to me meant that I would KNOW what I was talking about and that I would be educated in the nuances of healing.

What I didn't expect to gain was a journey of personal growth and experience that has left me virtually free of fibro symptoms for the last 5 years. I still get aches and pains, and my back still hurts, but for the most part I haven't dealt with the drama of fibro for most of the last 5 years. What a gift. I consider it a direct result of the work that I have done while working through the courses in the doctoral program.

Not everyone or even most people who have fibro are going to be able to take the time to get a Ph.D. as part of the journey of getting better. Most fibro patients are lucky to be able to read occasionally and to function outside of the fog now and then. What happened for me is I had to work in the store, and as long as I was there and it was so quiet (it took a long time for us to get customers!), I worked on the courses. I would never have been able to do this in a traditional job, but I worked in my own metaphysical wellness center and retail shop, so I had the luxury of lying down on my massage table for hours at a time when business was slow (usually!). Because I could lie down and ease my back pain, I was able to function in this job. If I hadn't been able to do this, I'm quite sure I never would have been able to improve.

My coursework started out with vibrational medicines like aromatherapy. That is a loosey-goosey feel-good topic if there ever was one and I was very resistant to the information presented. I thought it was really ridiculous that medicinal shifts could happen as a result of smelling things. I seriously doubted everything that was presented to me in this course, until I started using it as a result of one of the projects in the coursework. While I embraced the idea of energetic healing, the thoughts of vibrational medicine were a little bit outside my comprehension level. Eventually I tried the different vibrational medicines, but I was always a skeptic to begin with.

I believe lavender was the first essential oil that really caught my attention. I could see how it calmed me and relaxed me and really helped me to focus.

For many years I have had problems with scents and perfumes. They give me headaches and I avoided them at all costs. I learned through my aromatherapy class that it isn't really the scents that were causing the headaches, it was the additives. Armed with this knowledge, I cracked open my resistance a little bit and started playing around with the essential oils.

Essential oils are the deepest, purest parts of plants. They are distilled out of the plant using a variety of methods that bring the oils out in their purest form. In this form they actually have vibrational healing properties. Each plant has different properties associated with it. Lavender for example is calming and works as a sedative or to eliminate negativity. Bergamot is better for clearing. Tea Tree is very good for getting rid of deeply rooted ailments and for feet. The list goes on and on.

As I became more familiar with the oils, I began to make my own little concoctions. One of my favorites is my brain blend, which I created for the days when fibro fog was overtaking me and I needed to be able to think.

The only problem with the brain blend was remembering that I had it and then to take it. I finally put it by the cash register so I would see it constantly and not forget to use it.

As I went deeper and deeper into my course work I found my body responding and changing. The sound course was good for getting me up on my feet and moving, even just a little bit. It reminded me of the joy of music. I had always loved to dance and during the course we had to listen to different types of music with different beats. I had a tough time with this class because I am very sensitive to sound, however, doing the project I had to listen to a variety of music and document the affects that it had on me.

To my surprise, I found myself actually moving and dancing a little bit. I'd been bogged down by pain for so long I really didn't think there was any chance that I could move to music any more. I really had no desire to dance or to move. So, I experimented. I started with the music that used to make me happy. Prince's "Purple Rain" has a couple of great songs like "When Dove's Cry" that used to always make me fill up with joy. So, I put it on.

I found I couldn't sit in my chair. I had to get up and move. So I did. Not very much, not very long, but I got up and moved to the music. I felt a little spark of the old joy. I tried Toni Braxton's "Another Sad Song". Wow!!! That song makes me move. I took it out to my car. I put it in the CD player and watched my car vibrate. The vibrations in the car are no different from the vibrations between the music and my aura. In fact this is a really good way to demonstrate exactly how vibrations work. The vibrations that rock the car are the same vibrations (sound) that rock my soul. Not only do they make me feel better, but they heal my auric field and therefore my body.

This is a simple thing to demonstrate. Take a minute right now and put on some sort of music that uplifts you. It can be anything, as long as it makes your energy shift. Listen to it. Feel it. Know that there is something shifting in your soul. This is how it started to shift for me. This is the beginning of how I left my fibro symptoms behind.

Next time you think about it, play some music again. See how it makes you move, even if it is just tapping your foot while sitting on the couch. Movement is one of the big keys to getting your muscles work again. I know how difficult it is, but believe me it is worth it. Move your feet to the music. Do it again.

The next step for me was learning to breathe. How silly, you say... learning to breathe. I have done a lot of meditation classes and I know the value of abdominal breathing. But, how often do I practice it? Not very often, that's for sure. So, how to breathe? What difference does it make and why worry about it.

Breathing brings oxygen to all parts of the body. Of course it does, that's its job. But what does that mean? Oxygenated blood means that your cells get a little more of what it takes to make them function. When properly oxygenated, everything works better. Your muscles are more flexible, the bones are stronger, the pain shifts a little bit and (this is the key) your body relaxes a little. That little bit of relaxation helps to break the pain/tired cycle, so it is well worth the extra effort (very little effort) to breathe down into your abdomen, if only a few times a day.

For me this meant that I was better able to focus. Well, able to focus at all was a good thing so bringing the level up from 0 to maybe 2 on a 10 point scale was a huge deal. Today I function at or near 10 most of the time. When I don't, breathing is one of the tools that helps me to pull back out of my brain fog. It also helps me to relax and let go of the pain/fatigue cycle.

Here's how to begin breathing abdominally. Put your hand on your chest and your abdomen. Its ok, you can do it lying on the couch! Watch your hands move as you breathe. Which one moves? Usually it is the one on the chest. If you are breathing into your chest, you are not oxygenating your body. Close your eyes. (Ok, you can open them to read the instructions, but then close them again). Place your hands on your tummy, about 2 inches below your belly button (we also call this area the 2nd chakra). Now, imagine yourself breathing all the way down into your hands. Give it a try. Try again. It is difficult when you begin. Try again. Notice that when you breathe in, your belly expands. When you breathe out, it contracts.

Not only is breathing good for oxygenating your body and relaxing, it is also a way of meditating. Just this, breathing in and out, is the foundation for meditation.

Monks spend years learning to do this. Try for a moment, to just focus on breathing into your hands.

Wow, you say. I never knew it could be so hard to breathe!!! It isn't the breathing that is hard; it is getting our minds still enough to focus. That's the hard part.

Getting Back Into Life

So, here I was, breathing, moving to the music a little bit and smelling interesting smells. I believe, at this stage I had already made significant inroads in healing the pain cycle. I didn't know it of course, I just figured I was doing a handful of things that seemed to ease the depression a little bit and I didn't hurt quite as badly as I had before.

By now it was December, 2006. I'd been off work for about 9 months, had lost about 50 pounds and was still in a tremendous amount of pain every day. I took 5 Flexeril every day and several Relafen, to ease the pain. Nothing ever really removed it, but I found I was able to function a little bit with these medications. I think I had started to break the cycle, but it wasn't by any means gone, just a little better.

During the first 9 months of 2007 I worked through my Herbology, Vision, and Dreams classes. All of these had useful information, but none really transformed me like the sound and aromatherapy classes had. I continued working at my shop, plugging along through the days, losing a little more weight and sitting on the heating pad for hours on end. It seemed like I would never really be out of pain, although I had learned to live with it more or less.

In September, of 2007, I was at a holistic exhibition, where I was practicing Reiki and met someone who did "Quantum Healing". He put his hands on me for about five minutes, allowing me to heal my body using him as a catalyst. My pain was much less severe as a result of this encounter, and I really believe this is the point that began the process of letting go of pain.

By then my business partner had left, so I was the only person in charge and had to be at work most of the time. It was ok some days, but other days it was very difficult. I'd try to do invoicing and find that I couldn't remember what I was doing. In the middle of a project I'd try to match the inventory that came in with the invoice and would mess it up completely. I'd go back to it a few days later and try to straighten it out, but end up more befuddled half the time. There are some invoices I never did figure out and had to just let go of. Needless to say my books were not in the greatest shape!!!

One of the most important things that I learned about the healing process actually came to me in one of my last classes. It is the information about quantum healing and theories about holograms. These theories, which are explored in depth in part 2, indicate that every cell is a holographic representation of the whole and that healing work can be done at the outer levels of our aura to instigate change in our physical bodies. I don't want to go into too much depth in this part of the book, but in a nutshell, if you can heal the outside layer the inner layers are simultaneously affected. The other very critical piece to this is what heals the outside layer is vibrational medicine, which is also explored in depth in part two. Vibrational medicine is medicine that works on an energetic level to shift or act as a catalyst to the healing process.

Years later (after closing the shop and moving a couple of times) I find that the one symptom I still experience is that I'm limited in my endurance. I used to be able to do anything and everything, but these days, even without fibro pain, I still need to take it easy much of the time. I tend to over-exert myself when I feel good, which often results in far less energy the next day. I'm finding some balance, but it is a slow process. Other than this fatigue, I find that most days I am symptom free!

My Health Today

The next few months went by with less and less pain, until one day I realized that I had stopped taking medications except maybe once or twice a week. I certainly hadn't planned to cut down so much, but I've always been a big believer in less medication is better, so cutting down was very important to me. At this point I take what I need which is usually significantly less than 5 a month, instead of 5 a day.

I spent about a year and a half taking care of my father. His health declined at the same time I closed my business and lost my house. I needed somewhere to live and he needed someone to care for him, so we moved to Paradise CA together. Taking care of Dad involved lots of doctor appointments and running around. Although my health was much better, I could never have held down a full-time job.

After Dad passed, I seriously considered trying to work again. I started putting more energy into my photography business, which I've maintained, more or less, since 2001. I tried working a couple of craft shows, but soon realized I still don't have the energy to work a full day. My daughter had a baby, so I've moved to the east coast to help her take care of my grandson. Here, again, I find that I'd like to go to work again, but the energy required is beyond me.

My fibro symptoms are in remission most of the time. I can walk around the block, dance for a few minutes, go to a movie and play with my grandson. My quality of life is significantly improved from where it was on that March day in 2006 when I stopped working full time. As I mentioned, the one symptom that has not been eliminated is the chronic fatigue. It is significantly better than it used to be, but it still exists, especially on days when I do too much.

In the last year, I drove across the country three times. I drove from CA to MD when my grandson was born, drove home a few weeks later, and then drove out again, when we decided I would help take care of the baby. The trips across the country went pretty well as I allowed myself to stop when tired and didn't push too much on any one day.

I believe that breaking the pain-sleep deprivation cycle is the single biggest change that has helped me to be symptom free most of the time. If I over-do, I end up very tired and sometimes a little pain or fibro-fog creeps back into my life. I immediately go to bed and make sure that I ease up on my schedule. Managing this cycle allows me to live a rich, full life, which is far superior to my wildest dreams when I was in the throes of fibro. I encourage anyone else who has fibro to figure out a way to get enough deep sleep to begin to crack the cycle.

What Can You Do <u>Today</u>?

Many people with fibro or other chronic pain issues find it difficult to figure out where to begin to address the issues. My personal experience is that sleep and movement are two of the key factors in breaking the pain cycle.

Today you can start working on both issues. Getting deep enough sleep to find effective rest is challenging. For me, it took taking medication (acetaminophen and Benadryl) and buying a new bed and putting a feather bed on top of it. I love my bed and I keep it full of comfortable pillows and soft comforters. The feather bed makes all the difference in allowing me to sleep deeply without fear of adding to my pain levels. I am able to relax and melt into it.

Movement, the idea of movement, intimidates people with pain. We fear that movement will hurt us and believe that the only way to reduce pain is to be still. However, movement allows your body to heal so starting to move, no matter how difficult, is one of the keys to getting better.

My suggestion is you start very small. Find some music that stirs your soul. It can be something from your past that brings back a fond memory or it can be something new that catches your fancy. Turn it on, turn it up and allow yourself to move, just a little bit. Start by tapping your feet while sitting in a chair or on the couch.

If you don't want to or can't stand to listen to music, just move your feet a little bit. Turn them in circles, move them up and down. Do the same with your hands and head.

The smallest bit of movement and getting enough sleep can help you to turn the pain cycle around. It takes courage and it takes effort, but it is worth it to begin.

At some point add in a scent that makes you feel good. I recommend using an essential oil, or something else that is alcohol free, but gently add some great smells into your life. I keep a pumpkin spice candle in my room. I love the way it makes me think of the holidays, pumpkin pie and family. It always lightens my mood.

Don't overdo, don't spend a lot of money. Just move a little bit, allow yourself to sleep and find some great scents that bring up good memories. These little strategies can make a world of difference in your life.

Once you have started to move a little bit and have achieved a little better sleep add in things like yoga, meditation, walking or swimming. I highly recommend doing these at your own level. Even though I've done yoga for a while now, I always take the beginning or gentle classes because my body needs for me to take it easy. If you swim, make sure that you swim at your own pace, not someone else's. We know our limits and we know when to stop. Others might not realize our limitations. At the same time, stretch your limits, just a little bit.

I was terrified to begin moving and every now and then I go back to my fears. As long as I work at my own level and don't push too hard, I am always happy that I move. It helps ease aches and pains, gets the blood and oxygen circulating and clears my mind. I highly encourage you to do it, if possible.

The remainder of the book is actually my doctoral dissertation on chronic pain. It examines the different levels of the body and what kinds of remedies are appropriate for each level. Although it is based on very sophisticated theories, the information is presented in everyday language.

Part 2: The Research

Introduction

Fibromyalgia, like other chronic pain conditions, responds to a multitude of treatment options that resonate with healing levels ranging from the physical through the etheric and other bodies, to the spiritual level. Working to alleviate fibromyalgia symptoms and addressing root causes can be challenging and rewarding for both practitioner and the client. There are a multitude of options including those under the Western medical model, which work on the physical level, mainstream alternative options which can be effective at the physical and auric level, and vibrational healing modalities which work at the spiritual level.

The idea of healing on any level other than physical may seem odd, but the body has several layers surrounding it which are commonly known as the aura, which are the ideal place to initiate healing work. The auric field is comprised of several levels. The level immediately outside the physical layer is the meridian system. After the meridian system, working outward, there are the etheric, astral, mental and causal levels or bodies. While physical treatments are the one most readily recognized (because most people can see the physical body), the other layers have been recognized, photographed and otherwise proved to exist for many years. Each level has associated healing methods, although some of the methods work on multiple levels.

For example, at the physical level a practitioner might work with medications or massage. At the etheric, astral and mental levels, she would work with the meridian or chakra system and at the causal or spiritual level she would use energetic balancing or soul retrieval. Below is a chart from Richard Gerber's text, <u>Vibrational Medicine: The #1 Handbook of Subtle-Energy Therapies</u>, which outlines the various bodies and the methods of healing to which each level responds: **Multidimensional**

model of healing: (Gerber 317)

	Causal Body		Spiritual Healing
	Mental Body	Mental Chakras	Spiritual Healing
	Astral Body	Astral Chakras	Spiritual Healing
Magnetic Healing	Etheric Body	Etheric Chakras	Spiritual Healing
Magnetic Healing	Acupuncture Meridians		Spiritual Healing
Magnetic Healing	Physical Body		Spiritual Healing

At each level of healing, there are several options

for treatments. When dealing with the purely physical

level, the client may want to opt for what Gerber refers

to as magnetic healing. Healing in this manner, works

with balancing polarity rather than spiritual healing.

Other physical remedies include massage for pain relief,

swimming and yoga to get the muscles moving and

relaxed, or a variety of drugs to act as muscle relaxants

or as anti-inflammatories. Deep sleep significantly impacts the physical level.

Moving up into the etheric and higher levels, one might explore options such as balancing the meridians through acupuncture or Reiki, homeopathic remedies, gem elixirs, color therapy, flower essences or aromatherapy. When working at the causal or spiritual level, the practitioner usually focuses on vibrational medicine such as soul retrievals or energetic healing.

Each of these levels has a part to play in both the creation of fibromyalgia and the release of the symptoms. Working with each level to reverse the condition, frequently creates relief, often significantly.

What is Fibromyalgia?

Fibromyalgia is a syndrome, which has been recognized by the medical community since the early 1990's. Many people who suffer from the syndrome have sought medical treatment for a number of the symptoms, only to be told that there is "nothing wrong" because fibro is difficult to diagnose. The medical community eventually created the name fibromyalgia to describe the syndrome, which encompasses some specific symptoms. Fibro is diagnosed by eliminating other similar conditions and then through checking tender points.

In Your Personal Guide to Living Well with Fibromyalgia, the Arthritis Foundation indicates that the professional association for rheumatologists (ACR) has the following criteria for diagnosis:

- "History of widespread pain (on both side of the body, above and below the waist, present for at least 3 months)

- Pain in at least 11 of 18 "tender point" sites" (Arthritis Foundation 3)

According to Staud et al, in <u>Fibromyalgia for Dummies</u>, "people who have fibromyalgia say that they have at least several, if not all, of the following symptoms:

- Flu-like pain that can be severe

- A constant feeling of exhaustion

- Specific tender points that hurt

- Overall body aches

- Depression

- Muscle stiffness and pain

- Insomnia or other sleep disorders

- Extreme fatigue

- Mental malaise and confusion, often referred to as

  fibro fog" (Staud et al 10).

Along with these most common symptoms, people with fibro often experience other medical difficulties such as irritable bowel syndrome and chronic fatigue.

There are numerous theories about what causes Fibro, with many experts offering THE answer. The Arthritis Foundation indicates, "Scientists have not positively established any single cause for the disorder. Some researchers believe that an injury or trauma, physical or emotional, may affect the central nervous system's response to pain" (Arthritis Foundation 9). They go on to say, "there is an established link between fibromyalgia and depression, but no one knows if it's a cause of or effect of the ailment".

Similar information is found in <u>Fibromyalgia for Dummies</u>, which summarizes some of the theories,

"No one knows for sure what causes fibromyalgia, but physicians and other experts have come up with many fascinating theories to explain what might induce the onset of FMS. The cause could be hormones or autoimmune problems or biochemicals gone awry, or it may be related to a previous trauma, such as an injury that you incurred in a car crash or in another serious accident" (Staud et al, 11).

Staud also offers an alternative causes from Dr R. Paul St. Amand, who "believes that people with fibromyalgia build up caches of chemicals (phosphates) in their bodies. He believes that these deposits result in the pain and other symptoms that are characteristic of fibromyalgia" (Staud et al 121).

The theory that fibro could be caused by trauma is an intriguing one. From a vibrational energy perspective, problems or learning situations attempt to get our attention at the outer layers of the auric field, in the causal, mental, astral or etheric levels, prior to manifesting on the physical level. If a person cannot or does not hear or "get" the lesson at an outer level and it has to manifest physically, often the manifestation is some sort of traumatic event. If trauma is one of the causes of fibro (or any other illness) it is logical that the trauma would need to be relieved on all levels, not just the physical.

One of the key problems with fibro is that there is a complex pain cycle that is very difficult to break. Breaking the cycle is a major step forward in relieving physical symptoms. When a person is caught up in the pain cycle, he or she is often unable to sleep because the muscles are afraid they will be hurt or traumatized while sleeping. This lack of sleep makes the muscles more tired and therefore more painful, so the cycle perpetuates. Other fibro symptoms can easily be exacerbated by the pain cycle also.

Depression and foggy thinking can easily be traced back to lack of sleep. Depression, especially if anxiety is involved, can exacerbate the cycle of not sleeping and adding to pain. What is needed at this point is something to break the cycle at least at the physical level. For long-term relief or remission, it is highly likely that the trauma or origin needs to be addressed.

The Levels and their Interaction

The physical level or body is certainly the easiest to understand. It is easily seen, felt and part of everyday experience. From a Western perspective it is the only body that truly exists. Westerners are just beginning to embrace the idea that there is an auric field and within that field are other "bodies" which are just as real as the physical body but much harder for the average person to prove.

Just outside the body and truly interacting with it is the Meridian system, which is where the acupuncture points are located. The "acupuncture points on the human body are points along an unseen meridian system that runs deeply throughout the tissues of the body" (Gerber 122). Blockages in the meridian system link to dis-ease or illness. According to Gerber "when the flow of energy to the organs becomes blocked or imbalanced, dysfunctions of the organs occur" (Gerber

122). Stimulating the acupuncture points, removes the blockage and the client has the potential to return to health.

The etheric, astral, mental and causal levels are energy systems which are progressively further away from the physical body, moving toward the spiritual connection with the Universe. The outer bodies or levels are often referred to as the aura or the auric field.

People who can see auras can actually see the disruption (the lesson attempting to get our attention) in the auric field. According to Webster in Color Magic for Beginners, "When someone is healthy in mind, body and spirit his or her aura will literally glow with vitality. However, any dis-ease in these three areas is revealed clearly inside the aura" (Webster 80). People who cannot see auras can still see the effects of disruptions through Kirlian photography, which reads the energy fields around the body and translates the energy reading into colors.

The theory behind how illness manifests through these fields is that lessons for in this lifetime attempt to get a person's attention at the highest level. If they are not successful, and are not resolved at the higher levels, they will manifest further and further into the auric field, eventually ending up in the meridian system and then manifesting physically as blockages which are known as illnesses or dis-ease. It is possible to work with and resolve the lesson or the dis-ease at any level of the auric or physical field.

Although healing of the auric field has been done since the beginning of recorded history, the Western world focuses much more extensively on the physical body. In the medical world, applying Newtonian logic, this means that there is a physical problem that can be solved with drugs, surgery or other physical treatments.

Western society is now moving away from the restrictions of Newtonian logic and considering Einsteinian logic as it relates to healing. "The Einstein paradigm as applied to vibrational medicine sees human beings as networks of complex energy systems that interface with physical/cellular systems" (Gerber 39).

Barbara Brennan, in her book <u>Hands of Light: A Guide to Healing through the Human Energy Field</u>, delves deeply into Einsteinian logic regarding energy and how this logic translates into holographic and quantum healing. She sees the universe as an entire being, not as disparate parts making up the whole. "The whole universe appears as a dynamic web of inseparable energy patterns. The universe is thus defined as a dynamic inseparable whole which always includes the observer in an essential way" (Brennan 25). Her theory regarding humans as beings reflects this same logic.

Brennan indicates, "From the holographic framework of reality each piece of the aura not only represents but also contain the whole" (Brennan 26). The etheric body is a hologram or 3 dimensional map of the entire physical body. Based on evidence from multiple sources, it is clear that the physical body is a manifestation of the hologram, not the other way around. In other words, the hologram comes first, is a map of the body, and the body is created based on the hologram. "The hologram concept states that every piece is an exact representation of the whole and can be used to reconstruct the entire hologram" (Brennan 25). On a physical level one might consider how cloning takes place from a single cell. That cell has the blueprint for the entire body and the ability to create the whole being.

This relates to healing because it illustrates how any work done on the hologram itself will actually stimulate healing at the other levels. Each level connects to each other level through the auric field. If work is done at the spiritual level, it works down into the physical level via the other bodies. Working only at the physical level only solves the symptoms. Moving up into the higher vibrational levels allows the practitioner to work with, and frequently resolve, the actual problems that manifested in the physical condition.

The ability to work with the lessons or problems that created the physical condition (or the auric disturbance) occurs because the conditions are visible without regards to time and space. In the auric field "The phenomenon of the aura is clearly both inside and outside linear time and three-dimensional space" (Brennan 26). In other words, if a traumatic event or other significant disruption occurred early in the client's life, it is always accessible via the auric field.

Physical manifestation is a way to be able to deal with the lesson in a way that makes sense in this lifetime. "All measurements involving space and time lose their absolute significance. Both time and space become merely elements to describe phenomena" (Brennan 23). Fibromyalgia is an excellent way to work with numerous lessons simultaneously as physical, mental and emotional symptoms are all wrapped up into one syndrome.

Physical Level

Many people start seeking treatment at the physical level. They want to experience relief from the fibro symptoms, especially the pain, depression and "fibro fog". Working at the purely physical level there are a number of options including massage, swimming, yoga, meditation, chiropractic, heat, ice, and medications (over the counter and prescription).

Probably the most immediate gratification for pain and to help relax muscles is massage. Staud et al noticed "A study of the effects of massage on the painful areas of people with FMS revealed that subjects who received 14 massage sessions over the course of ten weeks received significant pain relief" (Staud et al. 154). It is important to note that massage on fibro clients generally needs to be much lighter than on normal clients as deep tissue work will seriously aggravate muscle pain for most fibro clients.

Along with massage, swimming in warm water has been shown to produce some muscle relaxation, if the water is warm enough. Swimming is excellent exercise, it doesn't exacerbate any of the symptoms and it allows the client to move his or her aching muscles, which will often provide some relief from aches. It is also great for increasing endorphins and alleviating depression.

Yoga, meditation, prayer, and Tai Chi, have all had success in helping with fibromyalgia symptoms. Each of the modalities helps to interrupt the pain cycle and can offer some relief if the patient is willing and able to utilize them.

At the purely physical level, yoga helps get the body to stretch and relieves some of the pain from not moving. Sometimes just getting a little movement going will help to alleviate the cycle.

Meditation is a phenomenal way to relax the body. "One study indicated that women with fibromyalgia who practiced daily meditation-about an hour a day for six days a week, over an eight-week period-reported lower levels of pain, better sleep , and lower levels of depression than when they'd begun the study" (Staud et al 189).

Prayer can be useful in that it takes the person's mind off of the physical problem and it also allows the person to accept their situation. "Prayer may act much in the same way as does meditation or Yoga, instilling calmness and an acceptance that you're really not in control, can't be expected to be accountable for everything, and you need not frantically rush about trying to solve difficult problems right away" (Staud et al 190).

Tai Chi has become much more popular in the Western world, especially for people who can't do high powered aerobics or other challenging fitness regimes. For a person with fibromyalgia it is a great way to get the body moving to break the pain cycle. "Tai Chi helps patients with FMS in two basic ways; the exercises are relatively easy to perform for people with muscle problems who find it difficult to perform more arduous exercises. Also, the exercises can help with relaxation, in a meditative sort of way" (Staud et al 174).

Chiropractic may be able to relieve some pain. According to Staud et al "Most ethical chiropractors will hope to give you significant relief and improvement in your pain problems, but they won't give you any guarantees that you'll be cured" (Staud et al. 162).

Heat and cold are useful in temporary relief. "Cryotherapy uses cold to dull or weaken your agitated nerve endings in the area being iced, making it harder for the pain signals to reach your brain" (Staud et al 149). Cold unfortunately also makes the muscles tighten, which can exacerbate the entire pain cycle, so for many, heat is a better choice. "Heat therapy may work much more effectively for you when you're in pain and need some relief right now" (Staud et al 151).

In dealing with the physical, medications may be recommended. Dr. St. Amand, who believes that phosphate buildups could be the cause of fibro recommends using Guaifenesin to relieve the pain. Staud et al. indicated "Dr St. Amand also strongly believes, based on personal and anecdotal observations of his own patients, that the regular taking of Guaifenesin can slowly rid the body of these chemical deposits [phosphates], and, consequently will eventually make patients with fibromyalgia feel dramatically better" (Staud et al 121).

There are several over the counter medicines Staud et al. recommend such as acetaminophen, aspirin, ibuprofen and antihistamines. While all of these can provide some temporary relief, it isn't likely that they will permanently relieve fibro symptoms. Staud et al.

indicate: "The simple short-term benefit of taking over the counter Tylenol is that it may give you some temporary respite from your widespread body aches and pains" (Staud et al 127). Adding an antihistamine may bring additional relief as well as allow the client to sleep, "...antihistamines, or "cold medicines" may give some people with fibromyalgia some (or even a lot of) relief from their overall aches and pains. The most popular examples are Benadryl and Tylenol PM" (Staud et al 129).

For working on the physical body there are a number of prescription medications that can also bring some relief, again mostly of pain symptoms. If breaking the pain cycle is the main goal, these might be appropriate. The most commonly prescribed medications include muscle relaxers and anti-depressants. Muscle relaxers can have the dual benefit of relaxing the muscles and acting as an anti-depressant.

"Flexeril is the most commonly prescribed muscle relaxant. This drug can also act as a mild anti-depressant because Flexeril increases the level of serotonin in the bloodstream" (Staud et al. 134). Flexeril can also work to interrupt the pain cycle by allowing the client to get some much needed sleep. "The sedating action of most muscle relaxants can help those FMS patients who have trouble sleeping to avoid yet another sleepless night" (Staud et al 135).

The flip side of this is also noted, "Often, people with fibromyalgia are taking antidepressants not for depression, but rather for their fibromyalgia. Research has demonstrated that low doses of some antidepressants, taken on a daily basis, can help block the pain of fibromyalgia or other chronic pain" (Staud et al 143). So, muscle relaxers can act as anti-depressants and anti-depressants can block pain.

The medical model tends to look at pain-killers, muscle relaxers and anti-depressants as the necessary ingredients for dealing with fibro, "Most people with fibromyalgia *need* to take prescribed painkilling medications, at least some of the time, in order to cope with the widespread pain and stiffness" (Staud et al 135).

Homeopathic remedies, aromatherapy, flower essences, gem elixirs, and color & sound medicine can all be useful to alleviate physical symptoms; however, they are also powerful at the higher levels. Each will be discussed in later chapters.

While medications may relieve symptoms, working with holistic alternatives focuses on eliminating the actual problem at a much deeper level. Holistic practitioners work with the client to eradicate the root cause of the condition. When working with a systemic syndrome such as fibro, this can be a challenging undertaking. There can be a multitude of root causes, including traumas, heredity, the person's sense of self, disruptions in the auric field etc. The most important tool is assisting the client to get in tune with her body and figure out the cause. Once the cause has been faced on the etheric, mental, astral, causal and spiritual levels, healing can occur on the physical level.

Meridian System

Traditional Chinese Medicine has utilized acupuncture for thousands of years. Acupuncture points are made up of a variety of lines which are directly related to particular organs within the body (i.e. gall bladder, kidney, or liver). The point of acupuncture is to unblock "chi" which is our life energy. "The acupuncture meridians are the conduit of energy flow that make-up this subtle energy network. The acupuncture points are the most physically accessible aspects of the physical-Etheric interface" (Gerber 204).

Through the acupressure points, practitioners are able to both determine what is wrong and by initiating treatment, they can unblock chi, "It has been demonstrated that the electrical characteristics of the meridians, as measured through the acupoints, contain important information about the status of the body's internal organs" (Gerber 204).

Even medical doctors who seem more dubious about "alternative" healing tend to grasp the benefits of acupuncture. Staud et al describe a study illustrating the differences between patients who receive real or "sham" treatments, "The patients who received the real acupuncture reported that they experienced significant decreases in their pain, while the women receiving sham acupuncture didn't have significant pain reductions. These effects lasted for about four months after the treatment ended" (Staud et al, 168).

Another way of working with the meridian system is by balancing the chakras through Reiki or other "spiritual healing" method. The chakra system is a series of energy "wheels" or vortexes, which spin in the energy fields at the etheric, astral and mental levels. The work in the higher fields moves into the lower fields and in the etheric field the chakras interact directly with the meridian system.

Although there are a variety of descriptions of the chakra system, it is clear that there are at least 7 major chakras, which work at the etheric, astral and mental levels. The chakras interact with the meridian system to assist the practitioner and client in diagnosing and releasing old patterns that cause dis-ease. In the book, Reiki for Beginners: Mastering Natural Healing Techniques, Vennells states, "Reiki works to achieve long-term improvements by helping the person address heal and release the issues that initially caused the problem" (Vennells 123).

Working at the meridian level is more effective than just working at the physical level. Many of the blockages are released and the body is able to heal symptoms. In the case of fibromyalgia, this could offer significant pain relief, although it would probably not heal the cause, which would be addressed at the higher

levels.

Etheric, Astral and Mental Levels

Vibrational medicines and quantum healing are utilized at the etheric, astral level and mental levels. While many of these medicines cross through the boundaries of each of the bodies, they work at higher energetic levels than just the physical realm and can actually help with cure rather than just relieve symptoms.

Vibrational medicines are forms of healing that do not necessarily have physical attributes that are "scientifically" easy to prove. For example, homeopathic remedies, gem elixirs and flower essences contain very little, if any of the molecular structure of the medicine that causes the response. For people steeped in Western tradition, it is difficult to believe the effectiveness of such small amounts of the remedies.

While this may be difficult to comprehend, there are a number of studies that prove the ability of a cell's memory to remain, and for the healing vibration to be effective, even though the actual cellular matter is no longer measurable. In his book, <u>Quantum Healing: Exploring the Frontiers of Mind Body Medicine</u>, Dr. Deepak Chopra discusses this phenomenon at length. It is summarized, "What is a cell, then? It is a memory that has built some matter around itself, forming a specific pattern. Your body is just the place your memory calls home" (Chopra 83). Brennan argues similarly, "Physicists found matter to be completely mutable, and on the subatomic level, matter does not exist with certainty in definite places, but rather shows 'tendencies' to exist." (Brennan 24).

Homeopathic remedies, gem elixirs and flower essences utilize the vibration from the cellular memory, which acts as a catalyst for change within the auric fields, the meridians and the physical body. According to Gerber, homeopathic remedies tend to be better at the physical level, however "Many homeopathic remedies can affect higher levels like the chakras and subtle bodies, but less often and less effectively than the other modalities. Also, certain gem elixirs (and homeopathies) are capable of affecting the causal and higher spiritual bodies" (Gerber 273). Gem elixirs and flower essences utilize the vibrational structure of a particular gem or flower's healing properties as a catalyst to assist the body in healing itself.

Sound therapy, color therapy and aromatherapy all combine work at the physical and vibrational levels. Each modality has some definite physical contact with the person, but reaches deeply into the vibrational fields. They are slightly different from other vibrational medicines as they are not altered, but are used in their original form.

Sound therapy can work in two ways. The sounds can evoke an emotional and/or physical response that allows the person to relax or perhaps to relive a memory or sounds can be used at the purely vibrational level to act as a catalyst to healing, with the sound waves energetically working with the person's chakra system and auric field. "I used it (sound) directly on the chakras to charge and strengthen them" (Brennan 241).

Colors heal in a similar manner. Blues tend to sooth while reds tend to charge a person. For example, a fibromyalgia patient might have a good response to orange, as it is associated with healing properties for many of the fibro symptoms. "Illnesses that respond well to orange include: asthma, bladder problems, bronchitis, chronic exhaustion, colds, depression, elimination problems, epilepsy, kidney ailments, lung problems, rheumatism, tumors and urinary problems" (Webster 81).

For fibromyalgia, finding the exact remedy or therapy can be a challenging prospect, simply because the patient feels so bad and probably has little energy to begin figuring out what to do. A simple start might be to find the most effective way to work with the depression and aches. This could be achieved with any one of the modalities, and could include a good aromatherapy mix to relieve depression and a homeopathic remedy to ease the aches.

Aromatherapy is great for helping to break the depression and/or pain cycle. In his book, <u>Aromatherapy Handbook for Beauty, Hair and Skin Care</u>, Erich Keller says, "Essential oils act upon the mood and various body functions through the sense of smell. The scent of the essential oils used in any preparation influences your spirit and physical well-being" (Keller 10). Even traditional doctors have seen the benefits of using aromatherapy, at least at the physical level, "Often thought of solely as a flavoring, peppermint oil can also be a mild painkiller to sore and tense muscles" (Staud et al 130).

As the initial layers are relieved, the patient may find that some of the deeper levels of the ailment are also being addressed. She may want work with a practitioner who can help her figure out how to get to the core of the underlying issues that caused the illness in the first place. She may want to move into quantum healing or some other sort of work with a practitioner at this point.

Quantum healing, a modality introduced by Dr. Chopra, is a method of inducing several levels of the body to work together to affect healing. He especially works with the energy from the mind (mental level) and physical body. In his words, "Quantum healing is the ability of one mode of consciousness (the mind) to spontaneously correct the mistakes in another mode of consciousness (the body)...If pressed for a shorter definition I would say simply that quantum healing makes peace" (Chopra 241).

In Quantum Healing, Dr. Chopra brings together meditation (awareness), sound therapy and bliss. Bliss is an interesting concept to bring into the healing world as it sounds very subjective and difficult to define. However, Dr. Chopra says, "Bliss is both objective and subjective. You can feel it as a sensation but it also affects measurable change- it can alter the heart rate, blood pressure, hormone secretions, or anything else for that matter. This is what allows bliss to be useful medically" (Chopra 228).

For a fibromyalgia patient, to experience bliss would be to allow her to work with her higher levels, in order to create physical change. "Quantum healing moves away from high-technology methods toward the deepest core of the mind-body system... you must get past all the grosser levels of the body-cells, tissues, organs and systems-and arrive at the junction point between mind and matter" (Chopra 18).

For a person dealing with the pain, depression and inability to cope with life, these alternatives offer some real hope for ending the cycle. Many of them can

actually touch the vibrational/spiritual level and heal the

root cause. The most effective methods of dealing with

the core issues are soul retrieval work and vibrational or

spiritual healing at the causal level.

Causal/Spiritual Level

Healing at the spiritual or causal or spiritual level means working with the energy, the trauma or the situation which caused the illness or dis-ease at its core. For many fibro patients, the root cause is directly related to some traumatic event. The goal then, is to re-visit the trauma and heal the wound. For patients whose fibro is based on early childhood or past life events, spiritual healing can assist the person in finding and releasing the patterns that initiated the cycle originally.

Healing at this level can be done using a variety of methods. Shamans use soul retrieval, some practitioners use Reiki, others use other hands on or off techniques that penetrate deep into the auric field and help the patient find the beginning of the pain. The method is not important, healing is.

Keith Sherwood, in his book Chakra Healing and Karmic Awareness discusses many of the problems that can manifest physically as a result of trauma, "Trauma can cause a loss of vitality, chronic fatigue, depression, anxiety, a loss of motivation, sexual dysfunction, creative blocks, and boundary problems" (Sherwood 255). Many of these symptoms are everyday problems for the fibro patient. In order to heal from the trauma a person must work on the energetic field, "A traumatic experience will have the most disruptive effect on the synchronistic function of human energy field" (Sherwood 254).

Sherwood indicates that the best way to heal from a traumatic experience is to bring in someone who can assist in dealing with the problem. "In order to overcome the effects of a traumatic experience, intrusions of qualified energy must be released and the ejected energy bodies and/or energetic vehicles must be recollected and reintegrated by a skilled practitioner" (Sherwood 255). A Reiki Master or other energy worker is frequently a good choice for releasing and re-integrating energies.

Reiki and other energetic healing modalities work with energy systems that are much broader than just the person's energy field. The reason these modalities are effective is that they tap into the energy field that connects all of us. "Reiki's main purpose is to improve the power and quality of our internal energy by 'plugging into' the Universal Life Force Energy" (Vennells 59). At this level, deep healing occurs, tapping into karmic or past life information, or traumas associated with the person's current or other present lifetime lessons.

Another phenomenon that often occurs as a result of trauma or perhaps as a precursor to other illnesses is the loss of part of a person's soul. Although this sounds very far-fetched to Western practitioners, Shamans have done soul retrieval work for thousands of years. In The Book of Shamanic Healing, Kristin Madden discusses soul retrieval as a term that is "commonly used denote the return of lost fragments of the spirit. The shamanic perception of this is that the soul can shatter or parts can splinter off due to some sort of trauma" (Madden 162). Shamanic healing exists as a partnership between the shaman or practitioner and the patient. The patient must be willing to fully participate in the process in order to obtain healing.

Shamanic healing and energy work both tap into the deepest part of the person's soul. They often bring up issues that are difficult to deal with and are very painful. Facing work like this takes courage and fortitude and the willingness to heal. Sometimes a person is ready to dive into this deep work immediately but more often the patient needs to have some foundational work done first. A person with fibromyalgia has probably been to many doctors to try to figure out what is wrong. Going to a shaman or an energy worker might be out of their normal realm, but these deep methods could just help the patient to obtain the healing they have been seeking.

Conclusion

The patient's willingness to heal is a huge part of any of this work. Many times people get caught up in the cycle of pain and forget or don't realize that they have a solution. "We can re-teach ourselves to be well if we are willing to look within for the answers and not hand over responsibility of our health to others" (Vennells 122). Sometimes there is a conscious payoff for not getting better, but usually it is not that simple. Usually the fibro or chronic pain patient has tried many options but has lost faith in the ability to get better. Often the only option seems like one more medication. Many times the patient doesn't even realize that there is a possibility to heal.

Healing at all the different levels of one's being takes a tremendous amount of courage and a clear decision to get better. Not everyone is cognizant that there ARE different levels, much less that these levels have a direct impact on their health. People who have fibro have been inundated with people who are sure they have the "right" cure or method for dealing with the pain or depression or fatigue. They have many cures for relieving the pain or depression, only to find that the new treatment can relieve symptoms for a time, but doesn't ever get to the root of the problem. Looking at alternative treatments may be a scary undertaking, but the results could be life-changing.

There is no one cure for fibromyalgia, but there are many alternatives for dealing with the symptoms and for some to get to the root cause of the syndrome. If a person is willing to get better, to participate in their healing and look into many alternatives, they may find that they are able to find relief. For some this will be a shifting of symptoms, but for some very brave souls healing the core issues is possible.

References:

Arthritis Foundation. (1997) Your Personal Guide to Living

Well with Fibromyalgia. Marietta, Longstreet

Publications.

Brennan, Barbara Ann. (1987) <u>Hands of Light: A Guide to

Healing Through the Human Energy Field</u>. New

York: Bantam Books.

Chopra, Deepak, M.D. (1989)<u>Quantum Healing:

Exploring the Frontiers of Mind/Body Medicine</u>.

New York: Bantam Books.

Gerber, Richard M.D. (2001)<u>Vibrational Medicine: The #1

Handbook of Subtle-Energy Therapies. </u>Rochester:

Bear & Company.

Keller, Erich. (1991). <u>Aromatherapy Handbook for Beauty,

Hair and Skin Care,</u> Rochester: Healing Arts Press.

Madden, Kristin. (2006) <u>The Book of Shamanic Healing.</u>

Woodbury: Llewellyn Publications.

National Fibromyalgia Association. (2011).

www.fmaware.org

Sherwood, Keith. (2005)Chakra Healing and Karmic

Awareness. Woodbury: Llewellyn Publications.

Staud, Roland M.D. and Adamec, Christine. (2002)

Fibromyalgia for Dummies. New York: Wiley.

Vennells, David F. (2007) Reiki for Beginners: Mastering

Natural Healing Techniques. Woodbury: Llewellyn.

Webster, Richard. (2006) Color Magic for Beginners:

Simple Techniques to Brighten and Empower Your

Life. Woodbury: Llewellyn.